HOMEMADE HAND SANITIZER

A Step By Step Guide to Make Your Own Anti-Bacterial & Anti-Viral Homemade Hand Sanitizers for A Healthier Lifestyle.

BY

Michael Cooper

DISCLAIMER

The information contained in this book is geared for educational and entertainment purposes only. Strenuous efforts have been made towards providing accurate, up to date and reliable complete information. The information in this book is true and complete to the best of our knowledge. Neither the publisher nor the author takes any responsibility for any possible consequences of reading or enjoying the recipes in this book. The author and publisher disclaim any liability in connection with the use of information contained in this book. Under no circumstance will any legal responsibility or blame be apportioned against the author or publisher for any reparation, damages, or monetary loss due to the information herein, either directly or indirectly.

Table of Contents

INTRODUCTION

CHAPTER 1: HAND HYGIENE

What is Hand Hygiene?

In healthcare settings, hand hygiene is the most vital ways of decreasing the transmission of infections. It's an activity that reduces the level of contamination with micro-organisms, like fungi, bacteria and virus etc. Hand hygiene includes handwashing, antiseptic handwash, alcohol-based handrub and surgical hand scrub.

Hand hygiene involves a way of cleaning one's hands to drastically reduce potential harmful microorganisms on the hands form gaining access to the body. It helps to reduce the risk of transmitting infection among patients and health workers. The procedures of carrying out hand hygiene involve the use of alcohol-based hand rubs which contains about 60%–95% alcohol and hand washing with soap and water.

For surgical purpose, do a thorough surgical hand scrub prior on wearing sterile surgeon's gloves. For routine dental and nonsurgical purposes, use an alcohol-based hand rub or clean water and antimicrobial soap. Once your hands are visibly soiled (e.g., dirt, blood, body fluids), an alcohol-based hand rub is recommended over water and soap due to the following reasons:

- It's very effective than soap at wading off potentially deadly germs on hands
- It needs a little amount of time
- It can be easily accessed handwashing sinks
- Produces reduced bacterial counts on hands, and
- It reduces skin irritation and dryness, thereby improving the skin condition.

Hand hygiene is one of the most effective ways of reducing nosocomial infections. **The U.S. Centers for Disease Control and Prevention** has proven that alcohol preparations containing between 60% and 90% ethanol or isopropanol decimates potential microorganisms better than any antimicrobial soap. After applying the hand rub to the palm of one hand, the hands and fingers should be rubbed vigorously to cover all the surfaces until they are dried. Hands that are soiled or visibly dirty should be properly washed with soap and water for about 15 seconds.

Why Should I Perform Hand Hygiene

It's extremely important to perform hand hygiene in the following situations:

1. Thousands of people die on a daily basis as a result of infections contracted while receiving health care.
2. Hands remain the major portal of entry for germs during health care.
3. Hand hygiene is the most vital measure to prevent the transmission of harmful germs and avoid health care-associated infections.

How Do I Perform Hand Hygiene?

1. You can perform hand hygiene by rubbing your hands with an alcohol-based formulation if hands are not visibly soiled. It is more effective than washing your hands with soap and water.

2. You can wash your hands with soap and water when your hands are not soiled or visibly dirty.

3. Wash your hands with soap and water when you have been exposed to potential spore-forming pathogens or outbreaks of Clostridium difficile.

Factors That Reduces Hand Hygiene Compliance

In a health care setting, workers' compliance with hand hygiene is reduced when there is patient overcrowding, understaffing and massive workload. In such situation, provision of personal alcohol handrub to be utilized by all health care workers that can make an impact on hand hygiene compliance rate becomes difficult.

Other reason that can lead to low hand hygiene compliance rate are when the health care workers are being too busy, skin irritation caused by handwashing and some workers prefer using gloves instead of handwashing.

Areas Of The Hands that Are Frequently Missed During Hand Hygiene

Areas of the hands frequently missed during hand hygiene are fingertips, thumbs and little finger. The right method or technique for performing hand hygiene should be demonstrated to all new healthcare workers and reinforced for existing staff through the use of hand hygiene posters, campaigns etc.

Methods of Hand Hygiene

Several methods of performing hand hygiene are:

- Routine handwashing with ordinary soap or antimicrobial soap and water for about 30 to 50 seconds.
- Alcohol-based handrub: this can be done by applying the handrub on the surfaces of the hands and remaining wet for about 15 seconds and then allowing to dry for about 40 seconds.
- Surgical hand decontamination with an antimicrobial soap and water at least 2 to 5 minutes.

How Does Hand Hygiene Reduce Infection Risk?

The physical activity of handwashing involves friction, rinsing and drying which helps to remove dirt and kill any potential germs from the superficial layers of the skin. Handwashing with the use of antiseptic products, like alcohol-based handrubs or medicated soaps helps to also kill or inhibit the growth of micro-organisms. By reducing the load of micro-organisms on a healthcare worker's hands through performing hand hygiene, the risk of infection transmission to the patient is reduced.

CHAPTER 2: HAND SANITIZERS

Hand sanitizer can be described to be a liquid or gel used to disinfect or sanitize the hands. It is a liquid or gel that is used in reducing or killing infectious agents on the hands. They are a specific type of antimicrobial agent that kill or permanently inactivate at least 99.9 percent of microorganisms when applied on the hands. The infectious microorganisms include viruses, fungi, and bacteria. Formulations of the alcohol-based hand sanitizer are more effective than hand washing with soap and water.

The alcohol-based hand sanitizers are more effective at killing microorganisms than soap and water. Hand washing should be done if your hands are visible soiled or following the use of the toilet. Outside the health care setting, hand washing is generally preferred when the hands is not visibly soiled.

Some hand sanitizers like alcohol-based use toxic chemicals as their active ingredient, so they can be dangerous when ingested. Hand sanitizers are often used in health care settings where there is an environmental risk of transmitting infection-causing pathogens, such bacteria, fungi and virus etc.

Types Of Hand Sanitizers

Alcohol-Based Hand Sanitizer:

These versions of hand sanitizers contain some combination of isopropyl alcohol, ethanol (ethyl alcohol), or n-propanol. The types that contain 60 to 95% alcohol are most effective. The alcohol-based hand sanitizers are most effective in killing microorganisms. Some alcohol-based hand sanitizers can cause dryness of skin. In such cases, you can use alcohol-based hand sanitizer with moisturizers. While, some varieties comprises of compounds like glycerol to prevent drying of the skin. Care should be taken when applying alcohol-based hand sanitizers because they are flammable.

In health care setting, alcohol-based sanitizers are usually preferred to handwashing with soap and water. They are more effective in killing microorganisms on the skin than repeated handwashing. However, some kinds of microorganisms like norovirus—are more effectively removed by handwashing with soap and water.

Alcohol-based hand sanitizers are very effective at killing many types of bacteria, such as MRSA and E coli, they're also effective at killing many viruses like influenza A virus, rhinovirus, hepatitis A virus, HIV, and Middle East respiratory syndrome coronavirus (MERS-CoV). They are not recommended for use on hands that are visibly soiled with dirt or grease. They have also found to be effective at removing certain types of chemicals, such as pesticides.

Alcohol-Free Hand Sanitizer

The alcohol-free hand sanitizers are free of alcohol but, comprise of quarternary ammonium compounds (usually benzalkonium chloride). These compounds have the tendency of reducing the activities of microbes but are less effective than alcohol. Alcohol-free hand sanitizer may not kill all types of germs, bacteria, & viruses.

They contain quaternary ammonium compounds (called benzalkonium chloride) in place of alcohol to reduce microbes. These agents are less effective in reducing the activities of microbes than alcohol. Alcohol-free hand sanitizers do not dry out hands because they create little foam after rubbing hands. Alcohol-free hand sanitizer contains 0.1% concentration of Benzalkonium, while the remaining solution contains mainly water & skin conditioner & vitamin E for moistening the skin.

How Does Hand Sanitizers Work?

Alcohol-based hand sanitizers kill germs by disrupting the membranes of various microorganisms, including many fungi, bacteria and virus etc. Not all viruses have external membranes. Viruses like norovirus cannot be killed by alcohol-based hand sanitizers. It's the virus that causes diarrhea on cruise ships.

However, coronavirus is not susceptible to being killed by alcohol and alcohol-based hand rubs. Hand sanitizers are effective in disrupting about 99.9% of germs. And one of those types of microorganisms it is likely effective against is COVID-19, which, as a member of the coronavirus, is membrane-enclosed.

How Effective Is Hand Sanitizers?

Centers for Disease Control and Prevention, recommended that the most effective way of fighting coronavirus is handwashing with soap and water and/or alcohol-based hand sanitizer. They categorically raised awareness to always "wash your hands with soap and water for about 15 seconds, especially after going to the bathroom; before eating; and after blowing your nose, coughing, or sneezing.

You can use alcohol-based hand sanitizers with at least 60% alcohol if soap and water are not available. Hand sanitizers are very effective in reducing microbes. Also, its important to wash your hands with soap and water and avoid touching your face.

Touching your face without performing handwashing with soap and water and/or using hand sanitizer is very dangerous because the microbes are transmitted via the mucus membranes of your face. Avoiding touching your mouth, eyes, and nose an extremely important preventive measure.

How To Use Hand Sanitizer

There are important points to be aware of when using hand sanitizer. You need to apply it in your skin until your hands are dry. And, if your hands are visibly soiled with greasy or dirty, then you need to perform handwashing with soap and water.

Bearing that in mind, here are tips to observe when using hand sanitizer.

- Apply or spray the hand sanitizer to the palm of one hand.
- Vigorously rub your hands together and try to cover all the surfaces of your hands and all your fingers.
- Continue rubbing for 40 to 60 seconds or until your hands are dry. The applied hand sanitizer will take about 60 seconds to kill all the microbes.

Pros And Cons Of Using Hand Sanitizers

Hand sanitizer should be place everywhere including offices, airports, malls, and most public bathrooms. It should be a must-have in your purses, bags and cars because it is safe and healthy to use.

The Pros Of Hand Sanitizer

1. **It Kills Germs:**

Alcohols have the ability to kill germs and bacteria. Hand sanitizer has the ability to reduce potential germs and pathogens as well as preventing the spread of viruses, fungi, bacteria etc.

2. **Accessibility:**

You can easily make use of hand sanitizer when you don't have access to soap and water. A small bottle of hand sanitizer can readily be available to use on the go. It can conveniently be carried in your bag, car etc.

3. **It's Cost Effective And Long Lasting:**

Hand sanitizers are not expensive and have a shelf life of 2-3 years. The smaller hand sanitizer bottles can last for weeks at a time with consistent use, while large bottles can last for months.

The Cons Of Hand Sanitizer

1. **Some Brands Are Ineffective:**

Some brands of hand sanitizers are ineffective because they do not meet the 60 percent minimum alcohol concentration required to effectively kill viruses, fungi and bacteria. So, it's very important to read the label to know what makes up the product.

2. **Can't Be Used On Grime:**

Hand sanitizer may be effective against germs, but it can't be replaced with handwashing with soap and water to remove any bodily fluids, grease, dirt or blood. When the hands are visibly soiled, they need to be washed with soap and water.

3. **Weakens Immunity To Germs:**

Frequent use of hand sanitizer may cause a resistance to both good and bad bacteria that can weaken your immune system in fighting off germs. Hand sanitizer should not be substituted with hand washing.

What Germs Can Hand Sanitizer Kill?

An alcohol-based hand sanitizer with the adequate alcohol proportion can quickly reduce the number of microbes on your hands. It can also help to kill disease-causing agents on your hands, including the novel coronavirus SARS-CoV-2.

However, some alcohol-based hand sanitizers have limitations and do not kill all types of pathogens. According to the Centre for Disease Control, hand sanitizers won't remove potentially dangerously chemicals. Hand sanitizers are not very effective at killing the following microbes:

- Norovirus
- Cryptosporidium (which causes cryptosporidiosis)
- Clostridium difficile (also known as C. diff)

Also, a hand sanitizer may not be effective when your hands are visibly soiled with dirty or grease. Your hands may be soiled after working with food, doing yard work, gardening, or playing a sport.

If your hands are visibly soiled, perform handwashing with soap and water, in place of a hand sanitizer.

Ingredients Required to Make Your own Hand Sanitizer

The following ingredients are required in making your own hand sanitizer ingredients:

- Isopropyl or rubbing alcohol (99% alcohol volume)
- Aloe vera gel
- An essential oil, such as tea tree oil or lavender oil, or lemon juice.

The effective hand sanitizer should contain alcohol and aloe vera in the proportion of 2:1. This will help to keep the alcohol content around 60%. It is the minimum amount required to kill most germs, recommended by the Centre for Disease Control.

How To Make The Most Effective Hand Sanitizer At Home

There are some very important points to consider when making your own hand sanitizers at home. Isopropyl alcohol is highly flammable. So, you should avoid it coming in direct contact with your skin because it will burn it. We enjoin you to use nitrile gloves as a general precaution. Once you're ready to get started, here's how to make your own effective hand sanitizer:

1. Pour the isopropyl alcohol and aloe vera gel into the bowl. Effective hand sanitizers need to contain at least 60% alcohol and the isopropyl alcohol and aloe vera should be in the proportion of 2:1. For every 4oz of isopropyl alcohol you add, you should mix 2oz of aloe vera gel.
2. Add essential oils to the mix if desired. It is not necessary to add the essential oils, but if you like a particular fragrance, you can add a few drops of oil.
3. Vigorously stir the ingredients with a spoon to mix and combine. Pour the mixture into plastic bottles using a funnel.

Key Points To Adhere To When Making Hand Sanitizers At Home

- Provide a clean space or counter. Wipe down counter tops with a diluted bleach solution beforehand.
- Wash your hands with soup and clean water before making the hand sanitizer.
- Mix the ingredients with a spoon and whisk together. Wash these items thoroughly before using them.
- Ensure that the alcohol to be used is not diluted.
- Give all the ingredients a good mix until they are well blended.
- Avoid touching the mixture with your hands until it is ready for use.

Is Hand Sanitizers Safe?

Hand sanitizer recipes should be kept away from the reach of children. Children may not be accustomed to using hand sanitizers, which could lead greater risk. The hand sanitizer recipes are intended for use by professionals but you can also make your own hand sanitizer if you properly stick to the guidelines.

Improper ingredients in hand sanitizers can lead to:

- Lack of efficacy, meaning that the sanitizer may not effectively kill the microbes.
- Improper usage can cause skin irritation, injury, or burns.
- Exposure to hazardous chemicals via inhalation.

CHAPTER 3: HANDWASHING

What is Handwashing

Handwashing is one of the most essential ways of protecting yourself and your family from germs and getting sick. It can also avoid people from getting sick with germs that are already resistant to antibiotics and that can be very difficult to treat. Handwashing can be regarded as one of the most important ways to prevent infection. You should learn when and how to wash your hands to stay healthy. Understand how to properly use hand sanitizer and frequent hand-washing is one of the best ways to avoid getting sick and spreading illness.

Preventing sickness by handwashing reduces the amount of antibiotics people use and can prevent about 30% of diarrhea-related sicknesses and about 20% of respiratory infections. Reducing the number of these infections by washing hands frequently helps prevent the overuse of antibiotics.

How Germs Spread

Frequent handwashing can keep you healthy and avoid the spread of respiratory and diarrheal infections from one person to another. Germs can transmit from one person or surfaces when you:

- Touch your mouth, nose, and eyes with unwashed hands.
- Eat or prepare food and drinks with unwashed hands.
- Touch a contaminated surface or objects.
- Blow your nose, cough, or sneeze into hands and then touch other people's hands or objects.

Key Times To Wash Hands

Frequent handwashing can help you and your family stays healthy, especially during these key times when you are likely to get and spread germs:

- Before, during, and after preparing food.
- Before eating food.
- Before and after caring for someone who is sick.
- Before and after treating a cut or wound.
- Before touching your eyes, nose, or mouth.
- After using the toilet.
- After changing diapers or cleaning up a child who just defecated.
- After blowing your nose, coughing, or sneezing.
- After touching an item or surface that may be frequently touched by other people.
- After touching an animal, animal feed, or animal waste.
- After handling pet food or pet treats.
- After touching garbage.
- After you have been in a public place.

Five Steps to Wash Your Hands the Right Way

Handwashing is easy to perform and it's one of the most effective ways to prevent the spread of germs. Clean hands can avoid the transmission of germs from one person to another and throughout an entire community—from your home and workplace to childcare facilities and health care settings.

Follow these five steps every time.

- Wet your hands in clean, running water (warm or cold), turn off the tap, and apply soap.
- Rub your hands with soap. Lather the backs of your hands, between your fingers, and under your nails.
- Scrub your hands for about 25 seconds.
- Rinse your hands well under clean, running water.
- Pat your hands dry with a clean towel or air dry them.

Diseases You Can Prevent Just by Washing Your Hands

Frequent handwashing can prevent you from contracting simple respiratory diseases to the novel coronavirus, this hygiene basic is the key to keeping you healthy.

1. Coronavirus

2. Norovirus

3. The flu

4. Pink eye

5. Salmonellosis

6. Mononucleosis

7. Hand-foot-and-mouth disease

8. Cytomegalovirus

9. Staph

10. RSV

11. Hepatitis A

12. Strep throat

13. Giardiasis

14. E. coli

15. The common cold

Where Handwash Facilities Should Be Placed

It's important to know the exact location of placing handwash facilities to encourage hand hygiene compliance. The following are examples of where handwash basins are needed:

- At the entrance of all wards and clinical areas.
- Inside each patient room.
- Inside all patient en suite bathrooms.
- Inside treatment rooms and physical examination rooms.
- Inside any room with a toilet.
- Inside or close to each nursing station.
- Inside each dirty utility room.
- Inside the dirty linen holding area.
- Inside or close to the staff lounge.
- Inside all isolation rooms.
- Inside the medication room.
- Inside any room where food is handled/prepared.
- Close to each laboratory work station.
- Inside each clinical laboratory and morgue.
- In areas where hands are likely to be contaminated like storage and disposal areas.

Handwashing vs Hand Sanitizer, Which Is Better?

It's important to note when to perform handwash and when hand sanitizers can be helpful, because it serves as the key to protect yourself from the novel coronavirus and other sickness like cold and seasonal flu.

Handwashing and hand sanitizers serve the same purpose of reducing germs. Handwashing with soap and water should always be a priority, according to the Centre for Disease Control. Only use hand sanitizer if soap and water isn't available in a given situation.

www.ingramcontent.com/pod-product-compliance
Lightning Source LLC
Chambersburg PA
CBHW081148020426
42333CB00021B/2708